EVIDENCE BASED

HEALTH TIPS

IMPROVE YOUR LIFE WITH THESE TOP EVIDENCE-BASED HEALTH AND NUTRITION TIPS!

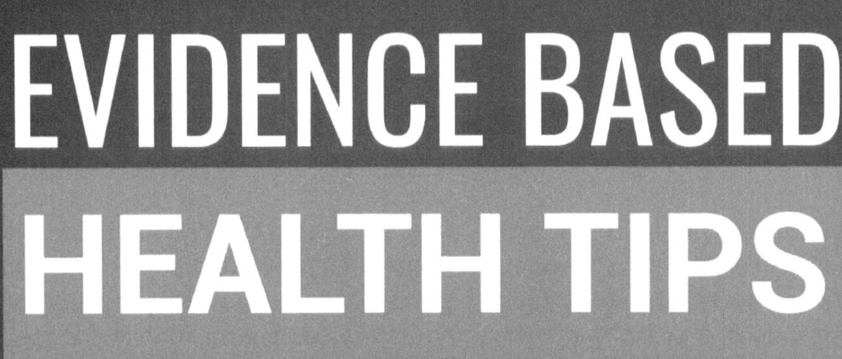

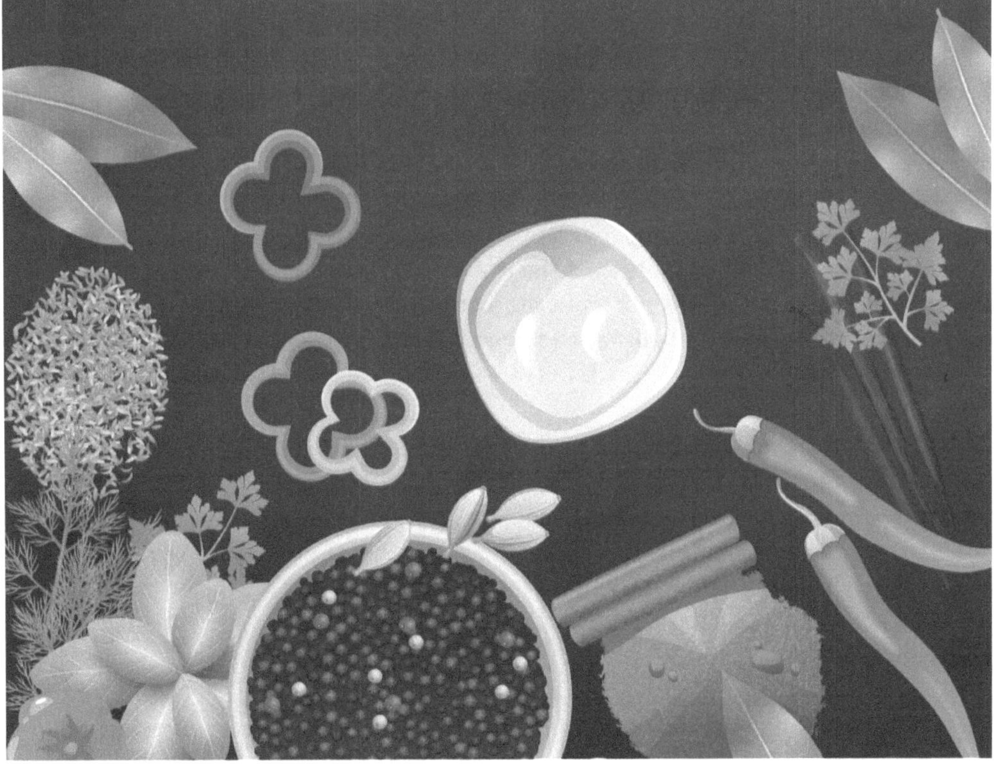

Table of Contents

Introduction

If you're looking to extend your lifespan, improve your overall health and look and feel your very best, you'll want to read **every word in this special report** dedicated to highlighting the **top evidence-based health and nutrition tips**.

When it comes to living your healthiest life, it isn't always easy to know where to begin. Even health professionals often have differing opinions in regards to what is considered healthy and what isn't.

That aside, there's a **ton of evidence** to support the following health and nutrition tips. In fact, all the information in this special report is based on **extensive research** rather than opinion.

That way, there will be no differing opinions because the information is based on extensive, time-tested research and not on some current fad or trend in the healthy lifestyle community.

Why is this so important?

Because when it comes to your health, the last thing you want to do is follow advice that isn't grounded in hard evidence. Instead, you should always base your dietary and lifestyle changes on **proven research.**

From what type of foods will improve your body's ability to self-repair, to the top nutritional tips that will help you live a vibrant, energetic and joyful life, you'll have all the information you need to live a longer, healthier life.

<u>**This includes:**</u>

- How to **immediately minimize your risks** of suffering from type 2 diabetes, obesity or high blood pressure.

- Top health tips to help you quickly get into the **best shape of your life.**

- **Important power foods** that will cleanse your system, **eliminating harmful toxins** so you can feel and look your best.

- And **much more!**

So, without further delay, let's get started!

You Are What You Eat

You've likely heard the saying, *you are what you eat*, and when it comes to living the healthiest you possible, no truer words have ever been spoken.

Quite simply, a healthy life begins with the foods you eat. What you put into your system ultimately dictates how you look and feel.

Makes sense, right?

A diet that consists of high-sugar foods, for example, isn't designed to sustain a healthy lifestyle. Those kinds of foods will rob you of energy and leave you feeling lifeless and bloated, not to mention the havoc it wreaks on your blood sugar levels and puts you at risk of many illnesses.

Start by thinking about how you feel after you eat certain foods.

Do you feel sick? Do you feel bloated? Are you tired? Run down?

Paying attention to the way foods make you feel is key in changing your diet so that it supports a stronger, healthier body.

Few of us analyze the way foods change the way we feel or affect our moods, but when we start to pay close attention, we discover just how easy it is to boost energy levels, improve our ability to focus and simply feel at our best just by eliminating these harmful foods from our diet.

Pro Tip: Consider creating a food diary or journal that documents the foods you eat. Start writing everything down for 30 days. After each meal, write down what foods you ate, portion size and how you are feeling.

Keeping track of how you are fueling your body, as well as how those foods are influencing how you feel both physically and mentally, is the first step towards identifying food-toxins so you can set yourself on a better, healthier path by eliminating them from your life.

Some of these foods may be obvious ones that you know are unhealthy while others may come as a surprise. Therefore, it's important to create a logbook of 30 days (minimum) so you not only have a detailed snapshot of how the foods you're eating may be impacting your health, but over the course of a month, you'll begin to develop a habit of considering healthier choices.

A food journal should also include a total calorie count so that you can reflect on the kinds of foods that are likely the leading cause of any weight-struggles you may have.

2 Foods to Avoid For Long-Term Health

When it comes to living a healthier life, there are a couple of harmful toxins that you'll want to quickly remove from your diet. These foods are notorious for wreaking havoc on our systems and leaving us feeling depleted of energy and unable to focus and thrive.

Worse, these foods ultimately increase our health risks in many ways, putting us in serious danger, so the sooner you can eliminate them from your life, the better.

1: Sugary Calories

It should come as no surprise that sugar wreaks havoc on your system. It can mess with your blood sugar and even with your brain since it doesn't quite measure calories in the same way it does solid food.

In fact, weight gain and heart health are just the tip of the iceberg when it comes to how toxic sugar is on your system.

Sugary drinks are also associated with type 2 diabetes, obesity and heart disease, just to name a few.

In fact, studies have shown that people who consume high-levels of fructose are in great danger of developing fatty liver disease because of the way excess sugar ends up stuck to your organs rather than being eliminated from your body.

Sadly, a report by the American Heart Association (AHA) discovered that the average American consumes approximately 22 teaspoons of sugar every single day rather than limiting consumption to only 6-9 teaspoons as recommended by health professionals!

So, by minimizing the number of sugary calories in your diet, you'll not only minimize your risks, but you'll eliminate a good portion of wasted calories: these are calories that don't provide nourishment or sustenance. They simply add inches to your waistline.

Need help getting over your sugar cravings? Here are a couple easy ways to get started:

Replace fruit juice with raw fruits:

Satisfy your sweet tooth and sugar cravings without risking your health by replacing fruit juice with raw fruits such as grapes or mangoes. Not only will they provide the sweet fix you're looking for, but they'll help stop sugar cravings in its tracks.

Eat Dark Chocolate:

When you're dealing with a sugar craving consider replacing high-sugar snacks with dark chocolate. Not only will this help curb sugar cravings but studies have shown that the antioxidant and anti-inflammatory compounds found in dark chocolate help improve your overall heart health!

Just make sure that you stick with chocolate that contains **more than 70% cocoa.**

So now you better understand the way sugar affects your body and the many reasons you should minimize your daily intake, but there's yet another common culprit hidden amongst our shelves and pantries and if sugar had an evil twin, this would be it!

Processed Foods

Processed foods are anything where there is some form of **chemical processing** involved.

While everything we eat is processed in some way, there's a difference between mechanical processing (such as in harvesting fruits and vegetables, for example) and chemical processing where unhealthy, artificial substances are injected into the foods.

These processed foods are loaded with all kinds of toxins, including sugar but they're also filled with dozens of artificial ingredients that you may not even recognize.

In fact, many of them have been carefully engineered to trigger pleasure sensors that provide temporary satisfaction while tricking your brain into overeating.

<u>Bottom line:</u> Processed foods are high in unhealthy ingredients such as preservatives, colorants and flavor chemicals, while low in important nutrients and proteins that your body needs to thrive.

Processed food can become just as addictive as sugar because it messes with your brain chemistry, hijacking your body's natural ability to detect when you're full. This leads to severe overeating and of course, that leads to obesity.

What We Learned from Harvard

Now that we've covered 2 of the greatest toxins, it's time to shift gears and focus on the foods we *should* be eating.

In 2011, **Harvard Health Publishing** released a visual health guide that focused on the healthiest foods on earth and how much we should be eating. They called this report, the *Healthy Eating Plate*; a detailed blueprint for healthy eating and portion control based on **scientific research.**

Here's just some of what they uncovered:

Increase your Fruits & Vegetable Intake

It should come as no surprise that most of us aren't eating enough fruits and vegetables, yet they carry some of the **highest levels of vitamins and nutrients** of all the food groups. In fact, the Healthy Eating Plate recommends that we fill half our plate with fruits and vegetables.

Some of the best fruits and vegetables are:

Spinach

This is a very nutrient-dense superfood and is one of the healthiest foods on earth. Spinach is loaded with nutrients and vitamins including Vitamin A, Vitamin K and essential folate, while being low on calories.

Beets

Beets are good for the heart and great for the brain. They're also excellent for lowering blood pressure! These powerful root vegetables are filled with Vitamin C, magnesium and folate.

Avocado

Consuming just 1-2 avocados every week will provide you with all the benefits of monounsaturated fats as well as loads of Vitamin B6 and folate.

Raspberries

Most fruits come loaded with antioxidants and raspberries are at the top of the list. Loaded with Vitamin C, iron and calcium they will provide you with a ton of nutrients while helping you curb those sugar cravings.

Lemons

Lemons not only carry powerful anti-inflammatory qualifies but they are proven to hinder the growth of cancer cells! They also offer tons of vitamins including Vitamin C, phytonutrients and folate.

Eat Whole Grains

Harvard Health Publishing also recommends that we fill ¼ of our plates with whole grains. This includes things like barley, quinoa, oats, brown rice and other whole and intact grains.

Healthy Plant Oils

When it comes to how we cook our foods, we need to be careful not to use unhealthy fats. Instead, swap them out for sunflower, peanut, olive, canola and other healthy vegetable oils.

And if you're a coffee drinker, you'll be pleased to know that coffee is healthy for you! Replace sugary drinks with water, coffee or tea. Just be careful not to load your coffee or tea with sugars or creams.

Healthiest Foods on Earth

We all have a good idea as to what we should and shouldn't eat. We've also been taught that a well-balanced diet is the key to a longer, healthier life.

But, what are the healthiest foods of them all?

It should come as no surprise that **kale** is amongst the healthiest foods available to us. Not only is it loaded with minerals, vitamins and antioxidants but kale provides our body with the natural fiber needed for optimum health.

Tip: Kale can be rather bitter so if you find yourself struggling to eat enough, consider putting it into soups or stews. Chances are you won't even notice it!

Next up, **garlic**. This is a food that we find in many of our favorite dishes, including sauces, roasts and stews and it's no wonder: not only does it add incredible flavor to our dishes, but it's loaded with Vitamins C, B1 and B6.

Then we have **seaweed**. This is an extraordinarily nutritious food, but it's not one that many of us consume on a regular basis so we'll have to look for ways to incorporate it into our diet. It's worth the effort though because seaweed is loaded with minerals like iron, calcium, magnesium and manganese, some of which aren't found in other fruits and vegetables.

Seaweed is also notorious for reducing inflammation because of its high levels of antioxidants!

Then we have **shellfish**. If you're looking to improve your overall health you'll want to start incorporating shellfish such as clams, crab, lobster or oysters into your diet because they're known as some of the best sources for vitamin B12 which impacts our energy levels and overall mood.

Note: They're also high in zinc, copper and Vitamin D, especially oysters so consider including them in your next meal!

Salmon is low in fat and calories but very high in protein which will make you feel fuller faster, helping you avoid over-eating.

Salmon is also known for its high levels of omega-3 fatty acids which have been proven to boost brain activity, improve focus and energy levels.

And even more impressively, salmon has been proven to prevent the onset of serious diseases because of its high levels of magnesium, potassium and selenium, important minerals that our body needs but never seems to get enough of.

And finally, we have **blueberries**. Not only are they loaded with antioxidants but they are high in phytochemicals which are linked to better brain function, such as improved focus and memory.

Live Your Best Life

We've discussed the different foods that you should work into incorporating into your daily diet, but increased longevity and optimum health go beyond what you're putting into your mouth.

One of the most important aspects of living your best life is to get plenty of rest.

We can't emphasize enough the importance of getting enough sleep. Poor sleep can boost insulin resistance, interrupt hormone levels and ultimately reduces both mental and physical performance.

Further, lack of sleep will put you at risk of depression and anxiety but it can also put you at risk of suffering a heart attack, high blood pressure, stroke and diabetes.

It can also age you rapidly. Lack of sleep will first affect your physical appearance, leaving you with premature wrinkling and dark circles around your eyes.

Over time, chronic sleep deprivation can increase your levels of the stress hormone, cortisol, which will break down collagen, reducing your skin elasticity and making you look twice your age.

Sleep is no joke. Make sure that you make it a priority to get enough sleep every night.

Not sure how much sleep you should get?

According to the National Sleep Foundation, who created a report based on two years of research, the average person between 36-64 years of age should be getting 7-9 hours of sleep a day.

Teenagers between the ages of 14-17, should get 8-10 hours of sleep and older adults, 65 years of age or older only need 7-8 hours of sleep.

Final Words

Living a healthy life starts with a well-balanced diet that includes the healthiest foods on earth. It also requires adequate sleep and of course, regular exercise.

Start by creating a lifestyle plan that includes a well-rounded diet. Consider planning your meals at the start of every week, including snacks. That way you can carefully plan in advance and avoid binge-eating.

Then, do your best to incorporate foods that are high in nutrients and vitamins while minimizing toxic foods such as sugar and processed meals.

Every high calorie meal you replace with a healthier alternative is one step towards creating habits that support a healthier lifestyle.

Take it one day at a time. Consider using a health journal so you can document your meals, exercise, and sleep pattern. Figure out what works best for you over time so you can begin to eliminate the habits and routines that cause you to get off course.

Don't beat yourself up if you make mistakes; we all do. It's impossible to always eat healthy. Sometimes life gets in the way.

The key is to do the best you can and to always be conscious of what you're putting into your body and how it ultimately affects your ability to feel at your best.

In no time, you'll be living your best life. A life where you feel and look at your very best.

You've got this!

Resources

Here are links to a few resources to help you continue your journey to a healthier and happier you:

Harvard Eating Plate:

>> https://www.hsph.harvard.edu/nutritionsource/healthy-eating-plate/

The Healthy Eating Plate guide, created by Harvard will make it easy for you to create healthy, well-balanced meals.

Health Line:

>> https://www.healthline.com/nutrition/50-super-healthy-foods

Health and diet resource that outlines the top 50 healthiest foods and provides daily tips.

Medical News Today:

>> https://www.medicalnewstoday.com

Free newsletter dedicated to living a healthy life. Includes articles and tips on improving your physical and mental health.

www.ingramcontent.com/pod-product-compliance
Lightning Source LLC
Chambersburg PA
CBHW051142250726
48655CB00007B/3195